CARB CYCLING FOR BEGINNERS

WOMEN EDITION

Copyright ©2023.

TABLE OF CONTENTS

FOREWARD

My name is Jane, and I have been struggling with my weight for years. I have tried countless diets that never seemed to last or produce the results I wanted. That is, until I discovered carb cycling.

Carb cycling is a diet where you alternate days of low carb and high carb intakes, depending on the type of workout you do each day. This diet has been a game-changer for me, and I have lost a significant amount of weight since starting it.

The biggest issue I had with dieting before was that I would get bored with the same meals every day. With carb cycling, I have so many different meal options, which have helped me stay motivated and on track.

My favorite thing about carb cycling is that it has taught me how to cook. I have always been a bit intimidated by the kitchen, but with the help of some amazing recipes from the internet and cookbooks, I have become quite the chef.

I decided to put all of the recipes that have helped me on my carb-cycling journey in a book, so that others can benefit from them as well. I have already sold a few copies, and the feedback has been great.

Carb cycling has changed my life in so many ways, and I am so grateful that I discovered it. I feel healthier, more energized, and I have even more confidence in myself. If you are looking for a way to lose weight, I highly recommend trying carb cycling.

INTRODUCTION

Carb cycling is a popular diet and fitness approach that involves alternating between high and low carb days. It can be an effective way for women to improve their health and fitness levels.

The idea behind carb cycling is to balance your body's energy levels by strategically using carbohydrates. On high carb days, you will be eating a higher amount of carbohydrates to give your body the energy it needs. On low carb days, you will be eating a lower amount of carbohydrates to help your body burn fat more efficiently.

By cycling through high and low carb days, you can create an optimal environment for weight loss and improved overall health. This approach can be especially beneficial for women, who may be at risk for certain health issues due to aging.

Carb cycling can help women lose weight and maintain a healthy weight, as well as improve their overall health and well-being. This book will provide a comprehensive look at carb cycling and how to effectively use it to reach your health and fitness goals.

We will explore the different types of carb cycling plans, how to create a carb cycling diet plan tailored to your individual needs, and how to tailor your carb cycling plan to your lifestyle. We will also cover different types of carbs and how to choose the right ones for your carb cycling plan.

In addition, we will look at the potential risks of carb cycling, how to stay safe while carb cycling, and how to make sure you are getting enough essential nutrients while carb cycling. Finally, we will explore how to maintain your carb cycling plan for long-term success.

This book will provide you with the information you need to understand and successfully implement a carb cycling plan for women. With the right plan, you can achieve your health and fitness goals and enjoy improved overall health in the process.

WHAT IS CARB CYCLING?

Carbohydrates are an important source of calories and energy for most people.

There are two types of carbohydrates: simple carbs and complex carbs.

Simple carbs contain one or two sugar molecules, while complex carbs have three or more.

Complex carbs include starches, such as cereals, legumes, and potatoes.

Carb cycling is a dietary plan where people alternate their carb intake daily, weekly, or monthly.

For example, some people may have a high carb and low fat diet some days and consume a diet low in carbs and high in fat on other days.

Carb cycling is a diet that people can modify to suit their needs. However, it may involve more planning than others.

In short, carb cycling aims to time carbohydrate intake to when it provides maximum benefit and exclude carbs when they're not needed

You can program your carb intake based on a variety of factors, including:

- **BODY COMPOSITION GOALS:** Some will reduce carbs during a diet, then add them back during a "muscle building" or performance phase.

- **TRAINING AND REST DAYS:** One popular approach is a higher carb intake on training days and a lower carb intake on rest days.

- **SCHEDULED REFEEDS:** Another popular approach is to do 1 or several days at a very high-carb intake to act as a "refeed" during a prolonged diet.

- **SPECIAL EVENTS OR COMPETITIONS:** Athletes will often "carb load" prior to an event, and many physique competitors will do the same before a bodybuilding show or photoshoot.

- **TYPE OF TRAINING:** Individuals will tailor carb intake depending on the intensity and duration of a particular training session; the longer or more intense the training is, the more carbs they will consume and vice versa.
- **BODY FAT LEVELS:** Many individuals will cycle their carbohydrates based on their level of body fat. The leaner they become, the more high-carb days or blocks they include.

BENEFITS OF CARB CYCLING

WEIGHT LOSS

As with any diet that restricts calories, carb cycling can help you lose weight in the short term.

There's one 2013 study, in particular, published in the British Journal of Nutrition, that shows promise. When 33 overweight women ate a carb-cycling-type diet for 3 months they lost about 2¾ pounds more and burned significantly more fat than their 27 counterparts who simply cut calories. Interestingly, both groups ate the same number of total weekly calories, but how they met that target differed: the carb-cycling group cut their calories pretty heavily just 2 days a week and ate "normally" 5 days a week, while the other group cut their calories by 25 percent every day.

However, it may not be the best long-term weight-loss strategy, as it can be challenging to maintain.

STRONGER MUSCLES

The high-carb days (also called "re-feeding") are also in place to refuel muscle glycogen, which may improve performance and reduce muscle breakdown.

IMPROVED FAT BURNING

The low-carb days are reported to switch the body over to a predominantly fat-based energy system, which may improve metabolism and the body's ability to burn fat as fuel in the long term.

BETTER BLOOD SUGAR

Another big component of carb cycling is how it affects insulin. Having low-carb days and targeting carbs around the workout may improve insulin sensitivity. This approach can help maximize the benefits that carbohydrates provide.

HOW CARB CYCLING WORKS

Carb cycling aims to help people with their weight and fitness goals by alternating between low and high carb days.

A diet low in carbs can offer a variety of benefits.

People who follow a low carb diet tend to consume more proteins and fatsTrusted Source that can make them feel full for longer. This also limits hypoglycemia, which in turn reduces hunger and calorie intake.

Diets high in nutrient-dense carb sources, such as vegetables and fruit, also have their benefits. Consuming meals high in fiber-rich carbs that include vegetables and fruits may reduce the riskTrusted Source of developing type 2 diabetes. Additionally, there is evidence that high carb diets increase insulin sensitivity in individuals with type 2 diabetes.

Eating fiber-rich carbohydrates may also lower cholesterol. This, in turn, may decrease the risk of heart disease.

The theory behind carb cycling is that people benefit from both high and low carb diets by alternating between these diets on a daily, weekly, or monthly basis.

THE SCIENCE BEHIND CARB CYCLING

There is some evidence that low carb diets help with weight loss and may speed up metabolism. Healthy high carb diets may also be beneficial because they reduce the risk of type 2 diabetes, heart disease, and intestinal cancer. While there are benefits to both nutritious high and low carb diets, there are few scientific research papers available on carb cycling.

CAN IT HELP YOU LOSE WEIGHT?

Anecdotally, carb cycling may be able to help people lose weight. However, there is currently no scientific research that suggests carb cycling is more or less effective for weight loss than other diets.

If people consume enough calories for their body weight, if they are a moderate weight, or have a slight calorie deficit if they have a high BMI, carb cycling may help them lose weight or maintain a moderate weight.

Research suggests there is no significant difference in weight loss between diets that restrict one form of macronutrient, such as protein or carbs, over another.

A study suggests diets that allow people to tailor food consumption and the type of food to their individual needs and preferences tend to experience better diet adherence and weight loss.

Carb cycling does not restrict a person's consumption of types of food as much as some other diets. Some people may find this approach more suitable for their needs and therefore may find this diet helps them with weight loss.

The National Institute of Diabetes and Digestive and Kidney DiseasesTrusted Source offer a free body weight planner, which may help people plan how many calories they consume in their carb cycling diet.

Carb cycling for muscle gain and sports performance

There is some evidence that low carb diets, such as carb cycling, may be beneficial for muscle gain and sports performance.

A study suggests that competitive bodybuilders who utilize carbohydrate refeeds, which are periods of times where they consume more carbs, do so because they believe it enhances fat loss.

Participants in the study stated that carbohydrate refeed days increased glycogen stores. They also noticed that these days aided their training performance and helped them mentally recover from their exercise regimes.

However, researchers need to conduct more studies to investigate the safety and effectiveness of carb cycling within the sports fitness community.

OTHER BENEFITS OF CARB CYCLING

There is currently no scientific research on the health benefits of carb cycling.

It is important to consume the correct number of calories for a person's daily requirements regardless of their diet.

It is also vital to consume enough macronutrients and micronutrients. Without sufficient quantities of these nutrients, an individual puts themselves at risk of developing undernutritionTrusted Source.

HOW TO CARB CYCLE

There are many variations to carb cycling, with people practicing programs on a daily, weekly, or monthly basis.

The amount of carbs that individuals eat per day will depend on whether they are consuming a high, moderate, or low carb meal. Examples of daily carbohydrate loads include:

- Very low carbohydrates: Under 10% of a person's daily calories will come from carbs.
- Low carbohydrates: Under 26% of a person's daily calories will come from carbs.
- Moderate carbohydrates: Between 26–44% of a person's daily calories will come from carbs.
- High carbohydrate: 45% or more of a person's daily calories will come from carbs.

EXERCISE PLAN FOR CARB CYCLING

1. **Cardio**: High-intensity interval training (HIIT) for 30 minutes, 3 times a week. Include exercises such as running, jumping jacks, jump rope, burpees, and mountain climbers. Aim for 20-30 seconds of intense exercise followed by 10-15 seconds of rest, repeated for 8-10 rounds.

2. **Strength Training**: Full body circuit training with free weights and body weight exercises for 45 minutes, 2 times a week. Include exercises such as squats, lunges, push-ups, pull-ups, and rows. Aim for 8-12 reps per exercise, with 2-3 sets per exercise.

3. **Core Work**: Core exercises such as planks, mountain climbers, and sit-ups for 15 minutes, 4 times a week. Aim for 8-12 reps per exercise, with 2-3 sets per exercise.

4. **Stretching**: Static stretching, yoga, or foam rolling for 15 minutes, 3 times a week. Focus on major muscle groups such as the quads, hamstrings, glutes, and lower back.

5. **Low-Carb Day**: Keep carbs under 50 grams per day, focusing on high-quality protein and healthy fats.

6. **High-Carb Day**: Increase carb intake to 150-200 grams per day, focusing on complex carbohydrates such as oatmeal, sweet potatoes, and brown rice.

7. **Low-Calorie Day**: Keep calorie intake under 1200 calories per day, focusing on nutrient-dense foods.

8. **High-Calorie Day**: Increase calorie intake to 1500-1800 calories per day, focusing on nutrient-dense foods.

9. **Carb Cycling**: Alternate between low-carb and high-carb days, 2-3 times per week.

10. **Hydration**: Drink at least 8 glasses of water per day.

11. **Sleep**: Aim for 7-8 hours of quality sleep per night.

12. **Stress Management**: Practice relaxation techniques such as mindfulness or meditation.

13. **Meal Planning**: Plan meals in advance to ensure adequate nutrient intake.

14. **Supplements**: Consider taking multivitamins and fish oil to ensure adequate nutrient intake.

15. **Activity**: Aim for at least 30 minutes of physical activity per day. This could include walking, jogging, biking, swimming, or any other type of activity that gets your heart rate up.

CARB CYCLING SAMPLE MENU PLAN

People can eat whichever healthy and balanced food they want on a carb cycling diet, as long as they do not exceed the amount of carbs their plan allows.

The following suggested meal plans are for people who require 2,000 calories per day.

HIGH CARB PLAN

Breakfast:

1 cup of cooked oatmeal served with milk and 1 cup of halved strawberries (51 g)

Snack:

1 serving of roasted chickpeas (22 g)

Lunch:

6-inch wholemeal wrap, half a cup of beans, 1 cup of raw peppers, grated cheddar cheese, and a medium apple (61 g)

Snack:

A medium banana and half a cup of skim milk (33.5 g)

Dinner:

1 cup of brown, long grain rice, 100 g of mixed vegetables, 1 serving of chicken, served with soy sauce (58 g)

MODERATE CARB MEAL PLAN

Breakfast:

3 large eggs, 2 slices of brown bread, 2 thick slices of tomatoes, 2 slices of bacon, served with butter (30.1 g)

Snack:

1 large apple (31 g)

Lunch:

3 ounces of salmon, half a cup of potato, and 3 florets of broccoli (14.8 g)

Snack:

1 medium banana (27 g)

Dinner:

1 portion of pasta with pesto sauce (26.2 g)

LOW CARB MEAL PLAN

Breakfast:

2 slices of bacon and 1 scrambled egg (1.2 g)

Snack:

1 large hard-boiled egg with 1 tablespoon of mayonnaise (0.7 g)

Lunch:

1 cup of chopped or diced chicken, 50 g of arugula, 1 cup red peppers, 1 cup of tomatoes, 1 cup onions, with olive oil dressing (20.9 g)

Dinner:

1 serving of shrimp, 1 cup of arugula salad, 1 serving of couscous, and salad dressing (25.4 g)

RECOMMENDED CARB SOURCES

While many foods contain carbs, there are some that people should eat more than others. Sources of complex carbs include:

- whole wheat cereals
- whole grain cereals and grains, such as brown rice
- wholemeal bread
- potatoes
- pulses, such as beans, lentils, and chickpeas
- vegetables
- fresh fruit

Carb cycling is a diet where people alternate between high and low carb days, weeks, or months.

This eating program may be beneficial for certain health and fitness goals, such as helping people lose weight, improve sporting performance, and increase insulin sensitivity.

CARB-CYCLING MEAL PLAN

DAY 1: Rest day, low carbs (30-50 grams)

- **Breakfast:** Greek Muffin Tin-Omelets with Feta & Peppers (7 g carbs)
- **Lunch:** Spinach & Artichoke Salad with Parmesan Vinaigrette (12 g carbs)
- **Dinner:** One-Skillet Chicken Paprikash with Mushrooms & Onions over riced cauliflower (12 g carbs)
- **Snacks:** Almonds, cheddar cheese, raspberries (5 to 8 g carbs)

DAY 2: Moderate workout, moderate carbs (100 grams)

- **Breakfast:** Apple-Cinnamon Overnight Oats (41 g carbs)
- **Lunch:** Mexican Spaghetti Squash Meal-Prep Bowls (25 g carbs)
- **Dinner:** Salmon with Curried Yogurt & Cucumber Salad over 1/2 cup cooked brown rice (30 g carbs)

- **Snacks:** Almonds, cheddar cheese, raspberries (5 to 8 g carbs)

DAY 3: Intense workout, high carbs (200 grams)

- **Breakfast:** Buttermilk-Oatmeal Pancakes topped with banana and syrup (101 g carbs)
- **Lunch:** Veggie & Hummus Sandwich (65 g carbs)
- **Dinner:** Pesto Ravioli with Spinach & Tomatoes (35 g carbs)
- **Snacks:** Almonds, cheddar cheese, raspberries (5 to 8 g carbs)

DAY 4: Moderate workout, moderate carbs (100 grams)

- **Breakfast:** Apple-Cinnamon Overnight Oats (41 g carbs)
- **Lunch:** Mexican Spaghetti Squash Meal-Prep Bowls (25 g carbs)
- **Dinner:** Sheet-Pan Sesame Chicken & Broccoli with Scallion-Ginger Sauce

over 1/2 cup cooked brown rice (34 g carbs)

- **Snacks:** Almonds, cheddar cheese, raspberries (5 to 8 g carbs)

DAY 5: Rest day, low carbs (30-50 grams)

- **Breakfast:** Greek Muffin Tin-Omelets with Feta & Peppers (7 g carbs)
- **Lunch:** Spinach & Artichoke Salad with Parmesan Vinaigrette (12 g carbs)
- **Dinner:** Shrimp Cauliflower Fried Rice (10 g carbs)
- **Snacks:** Almonds, cheddar cheese, raspberries (5 to 8 g carbs)

CARB CYCLING DIET RECIPES

LOW CARB CHOCOLATE PEANUT BUTTER BAR

INGREDIENTS

- 1 cup slivered almonds
- 1/2 cup unsweetened coconut flakes
- 1/2 cup natural peanut butter (no sugar added)
- 1/4 cup coconut oil
- 1 tsp vanilla extract
- 2 tbs cocoa, unsweetened
- 3 tbs monkfruit sweetener

INSTRUCTIONS

1. Combine slivered almonds and coconut flakes into medium bowl. Set aside.
2. Melt coconut oil and peanut butter together in small sauce pan over low heat. Whisk until combined.

3. Pour monkfruit and cocoa into sauce pan. Whisk until it creates a nice, glossy consistency.

4. Remove sauce pan from burner and add vanilla. Whisk again until combined. Let mixture cool while you line a baking dish with parchment paper. (9x9, or any size as long as you can divide recipe into 16 equal parts per nutrition info)

5. Next, pour the wet ingredients over the dry and mix together until well combined.

6. Pour mixture into the prepared baking dish. Smooth out the top with a spatula and add additional *optional* slivered almonds.

7. Refrigerate for 2 hours or freeze for around 30-45 minutes.

8. Once it has solidified, cut into 16 equal bars, serve, and enjoy!

SPIRALISED ZUCCHINI PUTTANESCA

INGREDIENTS

- 4anchovies, from a jar or tin, drained and chopped
- 1garlic clove, crushed
- ¼-½ tspchilli flakes or fresh chilli, deseeded and finely diced
- 2 tbspolive oil
- 200 gtinned chopped tomatoes
- 2 tbspcapers, rinsed
- 50 gpitted black olives, sliced
- 1 tspdried oregano
- 1large zucchini (about 200g), spiralised

INSTRUCTIONS

1. Over a gentle heat, fry the anchovies, garlic and chilli in the oil for 2-3 minutes. Press the anchovies against the pan with a wooden spoon to form a paste. Then add the tomatoes, capers,

olives and oregano, and cook gently for 20-30 minutes without a lid.

2. About 5 minutes before the sauce is ready, steam, microwave or boil the spiralised zucchini for 2-3 minutes, so that it is still slightly al dente.

HEALTHY LOW CARB EGG BREAKFAST MUFFINS

INGREDIENTS

- 1 bell pepper (your favourite colour)
- 3 spring onions
- 4 little cherry tomatoes/one normal tomato
- 6 eggs
- 1 handful spinach/ green leaves
- 2 slices cheddar (2 slices = around 50g; you can use different cheese too)
- ½–1 tsp salt
- 4–5 splashes hot sauce (or curry powder)

INSTRUCTIONS

1. Preheat the oven to 200°C/ 390°F.
2. Wash and dice the pepper, onions and tomatoes. and put them in a large mixing bowl.
3. Wash the spinach, lightly chop it and add it to the bowl as well.
4. Add the eggs and salt. Mix well. Pro tip – crack the eggs separately before adding. That way if you get a dodgy one, it won't ruin the whole meal.
5. Optionally add some hot sauce, curry powder…whatever you like. Hot sauce is great!
6. Grease the muffin tin with oil using a baking brush or Line muffin tin with paper muffin cups (I prefer using the paper muffin cups – less sticking and mess)

7. Pour the egg mixture evenly into the muffin slots.
8. If you're so inclined then layering some cheese over the top of each muffin before they go into the oven is a delicious addition! You can also mix in the cheese to the batter.
9. Pop the muffin tin into the oven for 15-18 minutes or until the tops are firm to the touch.
10. Cool on a baking rack.
11. Bon Appetit!!

SAVORY ROASTED ROOT VEGETABLES

INGREDIENTS

- 2 yams or sweet potatoes rinsed with skins on and chopped
- 2 red or purple potatoes rinsed with skins on and chopped
- 1 large red onion skins off, cut into chunks

- 1 cup Brussels sprouts rinsed and cut in half
- 2 large beets (red, orange or striped) rinsed with skins on and chopped
- 1/2 tsp Celtic or Himalayan salt
- 3 Tbsp fresh herbs (rosemary, oregano, sage, thyme) cut volume in half if using dried
- 1 tsp smoked chili pepper
- 2 cloves garlic crushed
- 2 to 3 Tbsp coconut oil
- olive oil extra virgin
- 1 bunch fresh parsley chopped for garnish

INSTRUCTIONS

1. Preheat oven to 450 degrees F
2. Place the cut vegetables, salt, herbs and spices, and coconut oil into a 9 X 13 inch baking dish and toss well using hands.
3. Transfer to the oven and roast for 45 minutes.

4. Let cool slightly and pour a swig of extra virgin olive oil on top.

5. Garnish with fresh parsley

ORANGE GLAZED BRUSSELS SPROUTS AND BUTTERNUT SqUASH

INGREDIENTS

- 1 pound brussels sprouts washed trimmed and halved
- 1 1/2 pounds butternut squash peeled then diced into 1/2 in cubes (about 3 cups)
- 3 tablespoons olive oil divided
- 2 teaspons coarse kosher salt
- [1 cup Sahale Snacks Valdosta Pecan Mix]
- Glaze:
- 2 tablespoons butter or ghee, melted
- 2 teaspoons honey
- 3 tablespoons fresh squeezed orange juice

- 1 tablespoon orange zest
- 1/2 teaspoon black pepper
- 2 teaspoons apple cider vinegar

SAHALE SNACKS VALDOSTA PECANS GLAZED MIX

INSTRUCTIONS

1. You have two choices. You can make the vegetables on the stovetop, or roast them! If you'd like to roast: mix squash with 1 1/2 tablespoons olive oil, and brussels with 1 1/2 tablespoons olive oil. Season with 1 teaspoon salt, each. Roast for 25 minutes at 400 degrees F.
2. If you'd like to make on the stovetop: In a large saute pan, heat 1 1/2 tablespoons olive oil over medium heat. Swirl to coat pan, then add in squash. Stir the squash pieces so they are coated with oil and sprinkle with 1 teaspoon salt. Shake the pan so squash

spreads out in an even layer and let cook, without stirring, so that they brown a bit on one side, about 5 minutes.

3. Stir and spread the pieces out again and let cook without

4. stirring so more sides brown. Cover, and cook about 6 minutes, until the squash is soft, but holds its shape. (This will depend on the size you cut your squash so try one to test.) Once done, remove from heat and pour into a bowl.

5. Heat remaining 1 1/2 tablespoons olive oil of oil over medium-high heat using the same pan. When it's very hot, place the brussels sprouts cut side down in the oil, sprinkling with 1 teaspoon salt. Turn the heat to medium, and sear on one side until nicely browned, about five minutes.

6. Turn the brussels sprouts over and cook on the other side until nicely

browned and tender, about five minutes. Some of the leaves can be charred dark brown or black.

7. Turn heat down to low and add the squash back to the pan, along with the pecan mix. If you've roasted, add pecan mix to the vegetables, removed from the oven. Mix all glaze ingredients together, and stir into vegetables, coating and warming through.

CHICKEN, ZUCCHINI AND POTATO SOUP

INGREDIENTS:

- 2 lbs. potatoes, peeled and cut into inch square pieces
- 2 lbs. chicken breast
- 2 lbs. zucchini, cut into inch square pieces
- 2 med. onions, chopped
- 5 c. low-sodium chicken broth

- 1/2 tsp. nutmeg
- 1 tbsp. per serving unsweetened Greek yogurt (optional)

INSTRUCTIONS

1. Place all ingredients into a crock pot, layering potatoes first, then chicken, followed by zucchini and onions last. Pour in low sodium chicken broth, and sprinkle nutmeg on top. Cover and cook for 8-10 hours on low heat. After cooking, shred chicken with a fork. When ready to serve, add a tablespoon of unsweetened Greek yogurt to each bowl and enjoy.

2. Maple Pecan Sweet Potatoes: This is another one of my favorite Chris Powell Recipes that actually Chris' wife, Heidi shared just after Thanksgiving. I love sweet potatoes and anyone who's looking for a Chris

Powell Carb Cycle Diet recipe to try should test this one out.

MAPLE PECAN SWEET POTATOES

INGREDIENTS

- 1/2 lbs sweet potatoes, cut into 1" cubes
- 2 oz pecans, chopped
- 1/3 cup 100% pure maple syrup
- 1 Tbsp butter, melted
- 1/2 tsp salt
- Juice of 1/2 lemon
- Pepper to taste

INSTRUCTIONS

1. Preheat oven to 400 degrees F.
2. Arrange sweet potatoes in a single layer in 9x13 inch glass dish.

3. Combine maple syrup, butter, salt, pepper and lemon juice in a bowl, and pour over potatoes.
4. Toss to coat and sprinkle pecans over top.
5. Cover potatoes with foil bake 15 minutes.
6. Uncover, stir and bake again, stirring every 15 minutes, until tender and starting to brown for 45-50 minutes longer.

CRANBERRY-QUINOA SALAD/STUFFING:

INGREDIENTS

- chicken sausages (I used sweet apple organic, but any vegetarian sub or tempeh would be great too)
- 1 medium onion, chopped
- 2 large apples, chopped
- 1\2 cloves garlic
- -5 C quinoa, rinsed and drained

- 3 C veggie or chicken broth
- 1 heaping T chopped fresh sage
- 1/2 t dried thyme
- -1/2 C dried cranberries

INSTRUCTIONS

1. In a large pan over medium heat, sautée the sausage, onion and apple in a little olive oil until soft, about 10 minutes. Add the garlic and season well with salt and pepper.
2. Transfer to the rice cooker (or if you want to cook it on the stovetop, a large pot)
3. Add the quinoa, cranberries, sage, thyme and broth.
4. Cook on the "brown rice" setting, or until light and fluffy (stovetop, cover and simmer for about 25 minutes)

5. It's a perfect lunch staple: on top of salad, or in a day-after-Thanksgiving style wrap with lettuce and cranberry goat cheese.

QUINOA AND BLACK BEAN STUFFED ZUCCHINI

INGREDIENTS

- 2 medium sized zucchini, about 10 to 12 inches long
- 2 tablespoons olive oil, divided
- 1 small onion cut in a small dice
- 1 medium sweet green pepper, cored, seeds removed and cut in a medium dice - about ½ inch.
- 1 cup [approx] fresh raw corn kernels [about 2 medium ears' worth]
- 1 cup cooked, rinsed black beans

- 1 large clove garlic, minced
- 1 teaspoon ground cumin [or more to taste]
- 1 teaspoon dried oregano
- 1 tablespoon hot sauce, like siracha or RedHot
- ½ cup red or white quinoa
- ¾ cup vegetable or chicken stock
- 1 medium tomato, cored and diced
- 1 tablespoon fresh, chopped cilantro
- 1 cup cheddar cheese, or a shredded blend, divided

INSTRUCTIONS

1. Start the broiler in your oven heating. line a large heavy baking sheet with foil [or not, if you don't mind a little scrubbing]
2. Cut the zucchinis in halves, the long way. Use a spoon to scoop out the centers, reserving for the stuffing, leaving a good half inch of flesh all around to form a stuffable "boat"

3. Brush about ½ teaspoon of olive all over the cut sides of the squash, and arrange the halves on the baking sheet, cut sides facing up.
4. Place pan with squash under the broiler - the rack should be adjusted to leave a couple inches space above the squash. Check frequently, and turn the pan so the surfaces brown evenly. You want some nice color, but the squash should still be fairly firm when you take it out. Leave the broiler on, as you are going to need it again in a few minutes.
5. Over a medium flame, heat a tablespoon of the olive oil in a large saute pan.
6. Meanwhile, chop the flesh from the squash, and add to the pan.
7. Add the onion, pepper, corn and black beans and stir fry for a couple minutes.
8. Add the garlic, cumin, oregano and hot sauce, and mix to combine.

9. Rinse the quinoa in a fine metal strainer [some quinoa can taste soapy if it's not rinsed.]
10. Add the quinoa and stock, and cover the pan.
11. Lower the heat a bit and cook until the quinoa is tender - about 15 minutes, adding additional stock or water, if things start to stick at all.
12. Remove the lid, and mix in the diced tomato, and the cilantro.
13. Mix in ½ cup of the cheese.
14. Portion the stuffing evenly among the browned zucchini halves [you may have a little stuffing left over], and top each one with ¼ of the remaining cheese.
15. Return the pan to the broiler for a couple minutes, until the cheese is melted and bubbly - watch carefully so that it doesn't burn.
16. Serve individual halves, or cut into slices for smaller portions. Can be

garnished with avocado, hot sauce, chopped cilantro and some sour cream if you like.

SKINNY PANCAKES

INGREDIENTS

- 2 egg whites
- 1/2 cup uncooked gluten-free oats
- 1/2 banana
- 1/2 tsp vanilla extract
- A dash of cinnamon

INSTRUCTIONS

1. Place all ingredients in a food processor or blender. Blend for 15-20 seconds or until mixed.
2. Spray hot griddle with non-fat cooking spray.
3. Pour batter onto griddle and cook until edges are golden brown. This should make about 3 small cakes.

4. Top with spray butter (if desired) and all natural syrup or agave nectar.
5. Enjoy!

CREOLE FLOUNDER

INGREDIENTS

- 2lbs flounder fillets
- 1 1/2cups diced tomatoes
- 1/2cup diced green pepper
- 1/3cup lemon juice
- 1tablespoon vegetable oil
- 2teaspoons salt
- 2teaspoons onion powder
- 1teaspoon basil
- 1/4teaspoon black pepper
- 4drops hot pepper sauce

INSTRUCTIONS

1. Heat oven to 450 degrees F.
2. Place fish in a greased 13" X 9" baking dish.

3. Mix remaining ingredients and spread over fish.
4. Bake 6-10 minutes or until fish flakes easily with a fork.

ROASTED SHRIMP, TOMATOES & FETA BAKE

INGREDIENTS

- 5 tomatoes, cut into eights
- 3 Tbsp Extra virgin olive oil
- 2 tbsp garlic, minced
- 3/4 tsp kosher salt
- 1/2 tsp freshly cracked black pepper
- 1 1/2lbs unpeeled shrimp
- 1/2 c chopped fresh parsley
- 2 tbsp lemon juice
- 1 cup feta cheese, crumbled

INSTRUCTIONS

1. Preheat oven to 450*
2. Place tomatoes in a large baking dish

3. Drizzle the olive oil over the tomatoes,
   add the garlic salt & pepper. Toss to coat.
4. Place on top rack of oven and roast for 20
   min
5. Remove dish from oven. Stir in the
   shrimp, parsley & lemon juice.. Sprinkle
   with the feta cheese.
6. Place back in the oven for another 10-15
   min or until shrimp are cooked. Serve
   warm with crusty bread.

THAI-INSPIRED YOGURT

INGREDIENTS

- 1 Tbspcreamy peanut butter, almond
  butter, or sunbutter
- 1 Tbspshredded Mexican cheese blend
- 1 tsphoney
- 1 tspsoy sauce
- 1/4-1/2 tspsriracha, to taste
- 1 CStonyfield Organic Greek Whole
  Milk Plain Yogurt or Stonyfield
  Organic Greek Plain Nonfat Yogurt

- 1/4 Cdiced cucumber
- 1small carrot, shredded
- 1 Tbsptorn fresh cilantro, fresh mint, or fresh basil (or all three)
- 1 Tbsproasted salted peanuts (or swap with cashews or sunflower seeds)

INSTRUCTIONS

1. In a small bowl, whisk peanut butter, juice, honey, soy sauce, and Sriracha until smooth. Add a little water, if needed, to loosen.
2. Place yogurt in a bowl and top with dressing, the remaining ingredients and any additional toppings, if desired.

CHOCOLATE WAFER COOKIES AND WHIPPED CREAM

INGREDIENTS

- 1 CStonyfield Heavy Whipping Cream
- 3 Tbspconfectioners' sugar

- 1 tspvanilla extract
- 1 CStonyfield Organic Greek Plain Nonfat Yogurt
- 19-ounce package of chocolate wafers
- 1garnish of your choosing (e.g. leftover wafer crumbs, grated chocolate, cocoa, raspberries, or cherries)

INSTRUCTIONS

1. Whip cream until thickened and then add sugar and vanilla. Continue to whip until soft peaks form; add yogurt and beat until stiff peaks form.
2. Assemble a stack by taking a heaping teaspoonful of filling and laying it on a wafer. Top with second wafer and gently press until about ¼ inch thick (the filling should be flush with sides of wafer). Continue until you have 5 wafers stacked. Finish with a dollop of cream/yogurt mixture. Repeat until you should have 6 or 7 stacks. Chill

stacks for at least 3 hours or overnight. Garnish with desired toppings before serving.

YOGURT INSTANT PIZZA DOUGH

INGREDIENTS

- 2 self-rising flour, plus more for dusting
- 1 cStonyfield Organic Whole Milk Greek Plain Yogurt or Stonyfield Organic Traditional Whole Milk Smooth & Creamy Plain Yogurt
- You Pick Pizza toppings of choice

INSTRUCTIONS

1. Combine flour and yogurt on a cutting board or in a bowl. Mix with hands until a shaggy dough forms. (The dough may appear dry and crumbly at

first, but it will come together as it's mixed.)

2. Turn the mixture out onto a lightly floured work surface and knead until the dough is smooth and slightly elastic, about 8 minutes, dusting with more flour if necessary.

3. Divide the dough in half. Use a rolling pin to roll out into two 10-inch pizzas. Spread out dough on non-stick baking sheets. Top the dough with your choice toppings. Cook until the crust is golden, 8 to 10 minutes, at 450°F.

STRAWBERRY CHEESECAKE ICEBOX PIE

INGREDIENTS

- 1 cStonyfield Organic Whole Milk Smooth & Creamy Plain
- 8 ozfat free cream cheese
- 3 Tbspsugar
- 1 tspvanilla extract

- 1 cstrawberries (diced
- 1graham cracker crust (9-inch)

INSTRUCTIONS

1. In a medium-size mixing bowl, cream together cream cheese and sugar.
2. Blend yogurt and vanilla extract into this mixture.
3. Fold in strawberries, and pour filling into graham cracker crust.
4. Freeze for 2-3 hours or until set.
5. Top with whipped cream if you like, and allow pie to warm slightly before serving.

YOGURT SHEET PAN PANCAKES WITH MIXED BERRIES

INGREDIENTS

- 1 1/2 cupsall-purpose unbleached flour
- 1/2 cupwhite whole wheat flour
- 2 Tbspgranulated sugar

- 2 tspbaking powder
- 1 tspbaking soda
- 1 tspkosher salt
- 1 1/2 cupsStonyfield Organic 0% plain yogurt
- 3/4 cupmilk
- 6 Tbspwater
- 2large eggs
- 2 Tbspunsalted butter, melted then cooled slightly
- 2 tspvanilla extract
- 1 1/2 cupsfresh or frozen mixed berries, blueberry, raspberry, blackberry
- Cooking spray
- Optional toppingsfresh berries, powdered sugar, maple syrup, honey or yogurt

INSTRUCTIONS

1. Move the oven rack to the middle position and preheat oven to 425 degrees F.

2. Spray a rimmed 18" x 13" sheet pan with cooking spray, this will keep the parchment in place.
3. Cut a piece of parchment paper to cover the bottom completely, about 16 x 20 inches. Place on the sheet pan and spray more oil on the parchment, and around the sides of the sheet pan.
4. In a medium bowl, whisk together dry ingredients (from flour to salt).
5. In another medium bowl, whisk together wet ingredients (from yogurt to vanilla) until thoroughly combined.
6. Transfer wet ingredients into the bowl with the dry ingredients and whisk until just combined. Do not over mix (or worry if there are some lumps).
7. Gently fold in berries.
8. Pour the batter into the prepared baking sheet. Spread the batter evenly with a spatula then tap the sheet pan on the counter a couple times to settle the batter.

9. Bake for 15 to 17 minutes, rotating the pan halfway through.

10.   Allow to cool for 5 minutes in the pan then, place a large cutting board over the top of the pan and flip the pancakes onto cutting board. Cut into 16 squares and serve immediately.

CACIO E PEPE FRITTATA WITH CAULIFLOWER AND LEMONY YOGURT

INGREDIENTS

- 12large eggs
- 3/4 cupfreshly grated Pecorino Romano or Parmigiano Reggiano, plus more for serving
- 1 1/4 cupsStonyfield Organic Whole Milk Greek Yogurt, divided
- 2 tspfreshly ground black pepper, plus more for serving
- 1 tspkosher salt
- 1small head cauliflower

- 2 Tbspextra-virgin olive oil
- 4 cupsbaby arugula
- 1lemon

INSTRUCTIONS

1. Preheat the oven to 450 degrees F.
2. In a large mixing bowl, whisk the eggs, cheese, ¾ cup yogurt, pepper, and salt until incorporated. Set aside.
3. Trim the cauliflower into florets; discard any tough parts of the stem. Chop the cauliflower into small pieces.
4. Set a large ovenproof skillet (preferably cast iron) over medium-high heat.
5. Add the olive oil; once it starts to shimmer, add the cauliflower, stir to coat, and let cook undisturbed for 3 to 4 minutes, or until it starts to brown.
6. Stir and cook for a few more minutes to increase the browning. Give the cauliflower one last stir and transfer the pan to the oven.

7. Roast until the it's browned all over, 6 to 8 minutes.

8. Transfer the skillet back to the stovetop (carefully; it will be hot!) and decrease the oven to 300 degrees F. This can be done ahead, or you can just pause and wait for the oven to cool down.

9. Set the skillet over medium-high heat.

10. Pour in the egg mixture and cook undisturbed for 30 seconds to 1 minute, or until the edges are just beginning to set.

11. Return to oven and bake the frittata until the top-center is just set, 25 to 30 minutes.

12. While it bakes, zest half of the lemon and combine it with the remaining ½ cup yogurt.

13. Season frittata generously with black pepper.

14. Slice warm, directly from the skillet, or wait for the pan to cool

down, set a large platter over the pan, and carefully invert it.

15.   Just before serving, toss the arugula with a bit of lemon juice (2 teaspoons or so).

16.   Serve slices of the frittata with about 1 generous tablespoon of lemony yogurt and top with the arugula salad; finish with black pepper and freshly grated Parmesan.

CAESAR-MARINATED CHICKEN KABOBS

INGREDIENTS

- 2anchovy fillets, finely chopped
- 1small garlic clove, minced or grated
- 1/3 cupgrated Parmigiano Reggiano
- 1/4 cupfresh lemon juice
- 5 TbspStonyfield Organic 0% plain Greek yogurt
- 1 Tbspextra-virgin olive oil, plus more if needed for the romaine

- 1 1/2 tspDijon mustard
- 1/2 tspfreshly ground black pepper
- 1 1/4 poundsskinless boneless chicken breast or thighs, cut into 1-inch cubes
- 8long wooden or metal skewers
- 1zucchini
- 1 large or
- 2 smallheads romaine
- 1/2 tspkosher salt
- Cooking spray

INSTRUCTIONS

- Make the Caesar marinade
- Add the anchovies, garlic and pepper to a large bowl and use your fork to mash into a paste.
- Add the cheese, lemon juice, yogurt, 1 Tbsp olive oil, mustard, and pepper and stir to combine.
- Reserve half for serving.
- Add the diced chicken to the bowl with the remaining dressing and stir to coat.

- Set aside to marinate at room temperature for 30 minutes or refrigerate overnight.

FOR THE KABOBS

1. If using wooden skewers on an outdoor grill, soak them in water for at least 30 minutes.
2. Trim the ends from the zucchini, halve it lengthwise, and cut it into semicircles between ½- and 1-inch thick.
3. Separately, cut the romaine in half (if using small heads) or quarters (if using a large head), leaving the root ends intact.
4. Lightly spray or coat the cut sides with oil.
5. Thread the chicken onto doubled skewers, alternating every few pieces with a slice of zucchini, for a total of 4 kabobs. Place the kabobs on a large

plate or baking sheet and, when they're assembled, season lightly with salt.

6. Preheat the grill with medium-high heat and oil the grates. Grill the kabobs for 6 to 8 minutes total, turning every 2 to 3 minutes, until the chicken is cooked through and well browned.

7. When the chicken is done, grill the romaine flat side down until it's lightly charred in places but still bright green and crisp, about 30 seconds per side.

8. Serve the romaine alongside the kabobs and drizzle the remaining marinade over both.

LOW-CARB BURGERS

INGREDIENTS

- 2 lb. Ground Chuck
- 1 tsp. Kosher Salt
- 1/2 tsp. Black Pepper
- 5 dashes Worcestershire Sauce
- 2 tbsp. Butter

- 1/4 c. Mayonnaise
- 1 tbsp. Dijon Mustard
- 2 dashes Worcestershire Sauce
- 2 whole Avocados, Sliced
- 1 whole Tomatoes, Sliced
- 1/4 whole Thinly Sliced Red Onion
- 1 head Iceberg, Green Leaf, Or Butter Lettuce
- Optional Toppings: Chopped Pickles, Feta Cheese, Cilantro, Pico De Gallo

INSTRUCTIONS

1. Make the sauce: Mix together mayonnaise, Dijon, and Worcestershire. Set aside.
2. In a bowl, combine ground chuck, salt, black pepper, and 5 dashes Worcestershire sauce. Form four patties and set aside.
3. Heat butter in a skillet over medium-high heat. Fry patties until done in the middle.

4. Top patties with tomato slices, avocado slices, and red onion slices. Drizzle with the sauce to taste.

5. Cut the base of each lettuce leaf on the head and carefully peel it away so that it stays as intact as possible. Use 2 or 3 leaves per burger patty and wrap them around the patty as tightly as you can.

6. Slice in half and serve immediately!

JAPANESE SALMON RICE

INGREDIENTS

• **Salmon** – Any salmon, will work for this, and for that matter, you could really do this with any type of fish that has a lot of flavor (though you couldn't call it Salmon Rice).

• **Salt** – I just used table salt to salt the salmon. If you use salt with bigger granules or flakes, you may want to increase the salt slightly to account for the volume difference.

• **Rice** – I highly recommend using Japanese short-grain rice for this dish. It has a higher ratio of amylopectin to amylose, which gives Japanese rice it's tender, sticky texture. If it's autumn when you're making this, look for "new crop rice." Freshly harvested rice has a sweet taste and tender texture that works perfectly for dishes like this.

• **Konbu** – Konbu contains a ton of naturally occurring glutamic acid, which is an amino acid that triggers the umami taste receptors in your mouth. When brought together with the cured salmon at the end, these amino acids have a synergistic effect, which cranks up the level of umami beyond what either of these ingredients would have on their own.

• **Sake** – Sake is another ingredient rich in glutamic acid and lends a mild sweetness to the rice.

• **Garnish** – I like to garnish my Japanese salmon rice with ikura to make Harako

Meshi, along with some mitsuba leaves, but if you can't find these, this rice is also delicious topped with a pat of butter and some chopped scallions.

INSTRUCTIONS

1. First, you want to remove any bones in the salmon with clean tweezers. If you don't have tweezers, you can remove the bones after the salmon is cooked, but I find it easier to spot the bones when the salmon is still raw. Now you want to slice the salmon, so it is about 1-inch thick. Too thin and the salmon will overcook, and if it's too thick, it won't cook through all the way.

2. Sprinkle all sides of each filet with the salt and then place them on a paper towel-lined rack set over a tray. Cover the tray with plastic wrap and refrigerate the salmon overnight. Once cured with salt, the salmon will keep

for about a week, so you can do this ahead of time.

3. For the rice, add it to a strainer and set the strainer in a bowl. Wash the rice until the water runs mostly clear.

4. Add the rice, water, sake, and konbu to a heavy-bottomed pot, like a dutch oven. This is important because we need a pot that can retain heat as the rice steams. Cover the pot with a lid and let the rice soak for at least 20 minutes.

5. Put the pot on the stove and bring it to a boil over high heat. Once it's boiling, turn down the heat to low and cook the rice for 12 minutes without opening the lid.

6. After 12 minutes, you want to turn off the heat and add the salmon on top of the rice. It's important to do this very quickly, or the temperature inside the pot will drop too much, and the salmon will not cook through. After the

salmon is in the pot and it's covered again, let this steam together for another 15 minutes.

7. When the rice and salmon are done, remove the salmon from the pot and keep the rice covered. Remove the skin and any remaining bones in the salmon, add the salmon back into the rice, and use a spatula or rice paddle to crumble and fold the salmon into the rice.

LOW CARB PROTEIN PANCAKES

INGREDIENTS

- 4 whole eggs
- ¾ cup egg whites (184 grams) (the equivalent of 6 egg whites)
- ¾ cup low fat cottage cheese (170 grams)
- 4 scoops Protein Powder (124 grams) (I used PEScience Gourmet Vanilla)

- ½ teaspoon baking powder
- Optional: 4 Tablespoons powdered peanut butter (like PB2 or PBFit) (24 grams)

INSTRUCTIONS

1. Place the ingredients into a blender in the order listed.
2. Blend until mixed together.
3. Pour batter onto hot griddle.
4. Cook until done on one side.
5. Flip and cook the other side!
6. Enjoy!

CONCLUSION

The carb cycling cookbook for Women provides an effective and sustainable approach to eating for weight loss and performance goals. This comprehensive cookbook provides easy-to-follow recipes, portion control tips, and practical advice for working carb cycling into your lifestyle. With its wide range of delicious recipes and helpful tips, this cookbook is an invaluable resource for anyone looking to start carb cycling. Whether you're a seasoned athlete or a novice dieter, this cookbook will help you achieve your goals and enjoy your food along the way.

All in all, carb cycling is a great way to eat for weight loss and performance goals. The carb cycling cookbook for beginners provides an easy-to-follow guide for anyone looking to start carb cycling. With its wide range of delicious recipes and helpful tips, this cookbook is an invaluable resource for anyone looking to start carb cycling.